DIVERTICULITIS DIET COOKBOOK FOR BEGINNERS

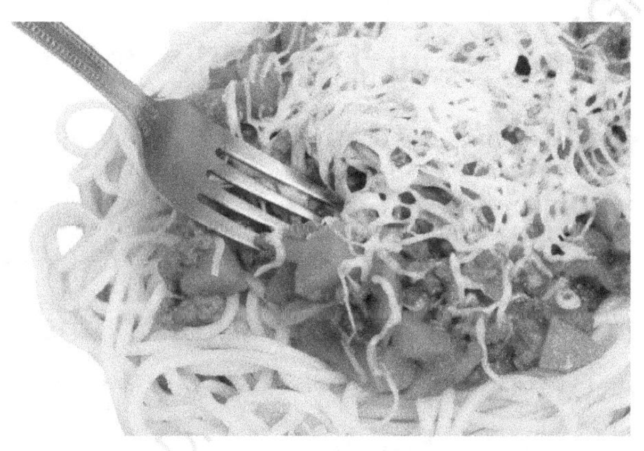

Guide to Overcoming Diverticulitis | Delicious Recipes with 21-Day Meal Plan for Managing Flare-Ups and Promoting Digestive Health

Dr. Kate W. Terri

Table of Content

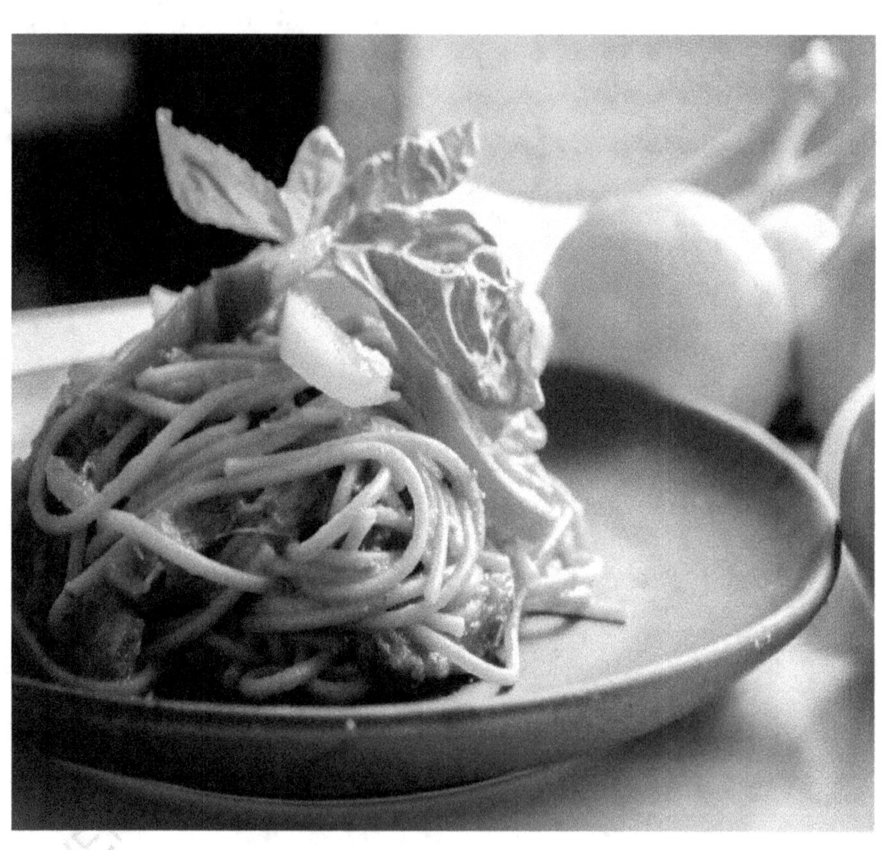

Introduction

Welcome to the Diverticulitis Diet Cookbook, your comprehensive guide to managing diverticulitis through carefully curated recipes and dietary strategies. This cookbook is designed for beginners who are looking to understand and implement a diverticulitis-friendly diet, ensuring a smoother, more enjoyable path to managing their condition. Whether you are newly diagnosed or have been dealing with diverticulitis for some time, this cookbook offers valuable insights and practical recipes that cater to your dietary needs.

Understanding Diverticulitis

Diverticulitis is a condition that affects the digestive tract, especially the colon. It occurs when small, bulging pouches, known as diverticula, form in the lining of the digestive system and become inflamed or infected. This can cause symptoms such as abdominal pain, fever, nausea, and changes in bowel habits. The exact cause of diverticulitis is not known, but it is believed to be related to a low-fiber diet, age, and genetic factors.

Key Points to Understand:

Diverticula Formation: These pouches can develop when weak spots in the colon give way under pressure, causing small pockets to protrude through the colon wall.

Inflammation and Infection: When these pouches become inflamed or infected, it leads to diverticulitis, causing significant discomfort and potentially serious complications.

Risk Factors: Factors that increase the risk of diverticulitis include aging, obesity, smoking, lack of exercise, and a diet low in fiber.

Understanding the nature of diverticulitis is the first step towards managing it effectively. By recognizing the symptoms and knowing the potential triggers, you can take proactive steps to manage the condition and reduce the frequency and severity of flare-ups.

The Importance of Diet in Managing Diverticulitis

Diet is essential for preventing and managing diverticulitis. The right diet can help reduce the risk of developing diverticulitis, manage symptoms during a flare-up, and maintain overall digestive health. Here are some key aspects of how diet impacts diverticulitis:

Fiber Intake:

Low Fiber Diet: A diet low in fiber can contribute to the formation of diverticula by causing constipation and increasing pressure on the colon. During a flare-up, a low-fiber diet is recommended to allow the digestive system to rest.

High Fiber Diet: For maintenance and prevention, a high-fiber diet is essential. Fiber helps keep the digestive system functioning smoothly by adding bulk to the stool and reducing pressure on the colon.

Hydration:

Staying well-hydrated is vital for digestive health. Water helps soften the stool, making it easier to pass and reducing the strain on the colon.

Avoiding Trigger Foods:

Certain foods can exacerbate symptoms of diverticulitis. Common triggers include nuts, seeds, popcorn, and certain fruits and vegetables with small seeds or skins. Identifying and avoiding these triggers can help you manage the condition.

Gradual Dietary Changes:

Abrupt changes in diet can be stressful for the digestive system. Gradual introduction of fiber and new foods allows the body to adjust and helps prevent flare-ups.

How to Use This Cookbook

This cookbook is structured to guide you through different stages of dietary management for diverticulitis, offering tailored recipes and advice for each stage. Here's how to make the most of this cookbook:

Start with the Basics:

Begin with the Introduction to each section to understand the dietary goals and benefits of each stage. This will help you make informed choices and understand why certain foods are recommended or avoided.

Try the Recipes:

Each recipe is designed to be easy to prepare, using ingredients that are gentle on the digestive system. Follow the recipes as provided to ensure they meet the dietary guidelines for diverticulitis.

Customize Your Diet:

Everyone's digestive system is unique. Pay attention to how your body reacts to various foods and modify your diet accordingly. Use the recipes as a foundation and feel free to modify them based on your preferences and tolerances.

Plan Ahead:

Use the meal planning and prep tips provided in the Special Considerations section to organize your weekly meals. Planning ahead can help reduce stress and ensure you always have diverticulitis-friendly foods on hand.

What is Diverticulitis?

Diverticulitis is a condition that arises when small, bulging pouches, known as diverticula, form in the lining of the digestive system, most commonly in the colon. These pouches can become inflamed or infected, causing diverticulitis.

The presence of diverticula is known as diverticulosis, which often causes no symptoms and requires no treatment. However, when these pouches become inflamed or infected, it progresses to diverticulitis, which can cause significant discomfort and complications.

Causes:

The exact cause of diverticulitis is unknown, but several factors are thought to contribute to its development::

Low-Fiber Diet:

A diet low in fiber is considered a major risk factor. Fiber helps to add bulk to the stool and facilitates its passage through the colon. Without sufficient fiber, the colon has to work harder to move the stool, increasing pressure on the walls of the colon. This pressure can lead to the formation of diverticula.

Aging:

The risk of developing diverticulitis increases with age. The colon walls tend to weaken with age, making the formation of diverticula more likely.

Genetic Predisposition:

Diverticulitis development may be influenced by genetic factors. Individuals with a family history of diverticulitis are more likely to develop the condition themselves.
Obesity:

Being overweight increases the risk of diverticulitis. Excess body weight, particularly around the abdomen, can put additional pressure on the colon.

Lack of Exercise:

Regular physical activity helps maintain healthy bowel movements. A sedentary lifestyle can contribute to constipation and increased colon pressure, leading to diverticula formation.

Smoking:

Smoking has been linked to a higher risk of diverticuliti. The harmful effects of smoking may affect the colon's health and function.
Certain Medications:

The use of certain medications, such as nonsteroidal anti-inflammatory drugs (NSAIDs), steroids, and opioids, can increase the risk of diverticulitis by affecting the integrity and function of the colon.

Symptoms:

The symptoms of diverticulitis can vary in severity and may include:

Abdominal Pain:

The most common symptom is pain, often in the lower left side of the abdomen. The pain can be severe and persistent, and it may worsen with movement or pressure.

Fever:

A low-grade fever is a common sign of inflammation or infection.

Nausea and Vomiting:

Inflammation or infection can cause nausea and vomiting.

Changes in Bowel Habits:

Diverticulitis can alter bowel habits, resulting in constipation or diarrhea.
Bloating and Gas:

Common symptoms include abdominal bloating and excess gas.
Loss of Appetite:

Pain and discomfort can lead to a reduced appetite.

Rectal Bleeding:

In some cases, diverticulitis can cause bleeding in the colon, leading to blood in the stool.

Diverticulitis is typically diagnosed using a medical history, physical examination, and diagnostic tests:

Medical History:

The doctor will review the patient's medical history, symptoms, and risk factors to identify potential diverticulitis.

Physical Examination:

A physical exam, including pressing on the abdomen to check for tenderness and pain, helps assess the location and severity of the inflammation.

Blood Tests:

Blood tests can check for signs of infection or inflammation, such as an elevated white blood cell count.

Imaging Tests:

Imaging tests, such as a CT scan, are commonly used to confirm the diagnosis of diverticulitis. A CT scan provides detailed images of the colon, allowing the doctor to identify inflamed or infected diverticula.

Stool Tests:

Stool tests may be conducted to rule out other causes of abdominal pain and to check for the presence of blood or infections.

Diverticulitis is treated based on its severity. It can range from conservative management with diet and medication to surgical intervention in severe cases.

Conservative Treatment

Dietary Modifications:

During an acute flare-up, a clear liquid diet is often recommended to rest the colon. Gradually, a low-fiber diet is introduced until the symptoms improve. Once recovery begins, a high-fiber diet is advised to prevent future episodes.

Medications:

Antibiotics may be prescribed to treat infection. Pain relievers, such as acetaminophen, can help manage pain. NSAIDs are generally avoided due to their potential to worsen symptoms.

Rest and Hydration:

Bed rest and adequate hydration are essential during an acute episode to allow the body to heal.

Surgical Treatment

In severe cases or when complications arise, surgery may be necessary. Surgical options include:

Bowel Resection:

Removing the affected portion of the colon and rejoining the healthy sections. This is often done to prevent recurrent episodes and complications.

Abscess Drainage:

If an abscess forms, it may need to be drained surgically or through a needle guided by imaging techniques.

Emergency Surgery:

In cases of perforation, severe infection, or obstruction, emergency surgery is required to address the life-threatening complications.

Long-Term Management

High-Fiber Diet:

After recovery from an acute episode, maintaining a high-fiber diet is crucial to prevent future flare-ups. Foods rich in fiber, such as fruits, vegetables, whole grains, and legumes, help keep the digestive system functioning smoothly.

Regular Exercise:

Regular physical activity helps promote healthy bowel movements and reduces the risk of constipation.

Hydration:

Drinking plenty of water is essential to keep the stool soft and easy to pass.

Avoiding Triggers:

Identifying and avoiding foods that trigger symptoms can help manage the condition. This may include certain seeds, nuts, and processed foods.

Regular Medical Check-Ups:

Regular follow-ups with a healthcare provider can help monitor the condition and prevent complications.

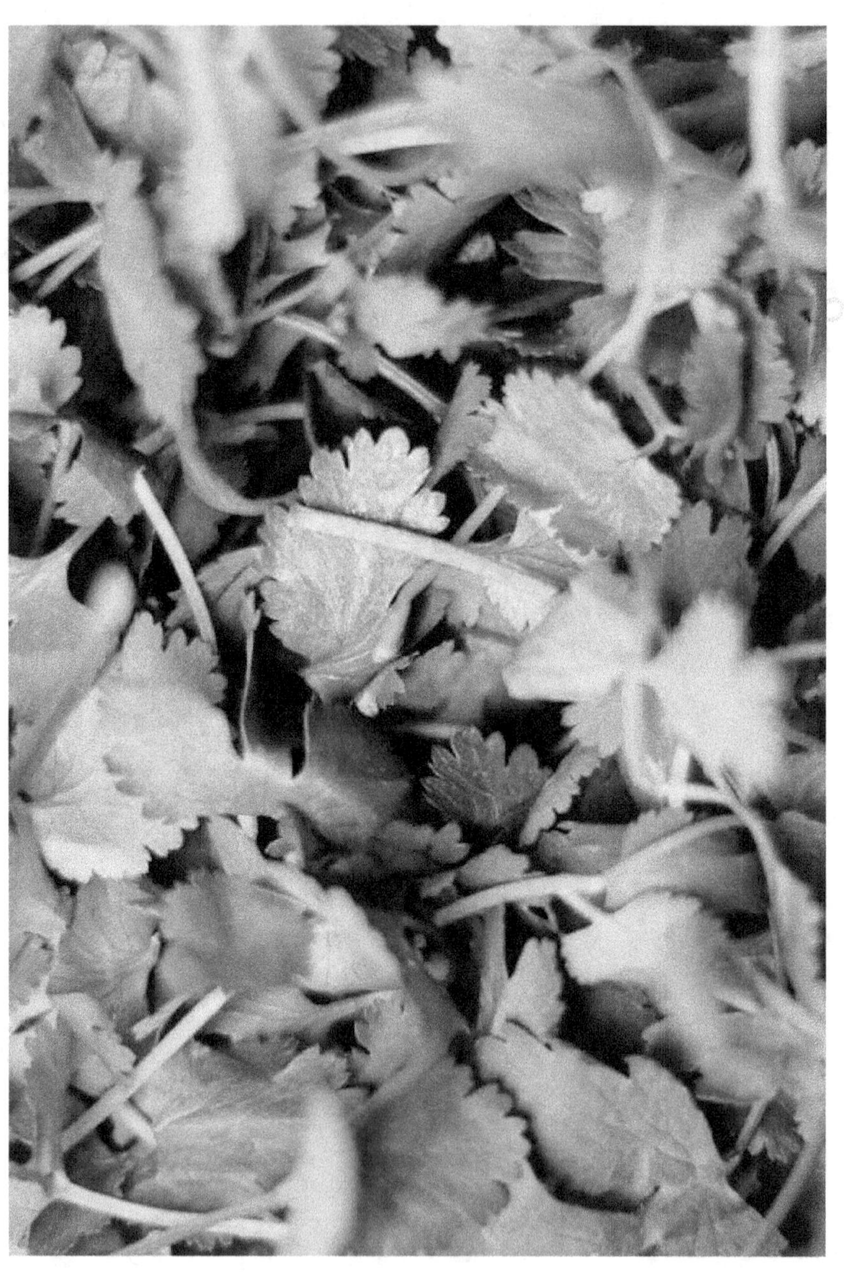

The Diverticulitis Diet

The Diverticulitis Diet is a dietary approach designed to manage and prevent the symptoms of diverticulitis, a condition characterized by the inflammation or infection of small pouches (diverticula) in the colon. The diet focuses on reducing inflammation, promoting healing during flare-ups, and maintaining overall digestive health to prevent future episodes. It typically involves different stages that correspond to the severity of symptoms, starting with a clear liquid diet during acute flare-ups and progressing to a high-fiber diet for long-term management.

Stages of the Diet

The Diverticulitis Diet can be divided into three primary stages: the Clear Liquid Diet, the Low Fiber Diet, and the High Fiber Diet. Each stage has specific dietary goals and recommendations to support the healing process and maintain digestive health.

Clear Liquid Diet:

Purpose:

The clear liquid diet is recommended during acute flare-ups of diverticulitis. The goal is to give the colon a chance to rest and heal by minimizing digestive activity.

Allowed Foods:

- Clear broths (chicken, beef, or vegetable)

- Clear juices (without pulp) such as apple or white grape juice
- Gelatin (without fruit pieces or other additions)
- Herbal teas (without caffeine)
- Water and electrolyte drinks
- Ice pops without fruit pieces or cream

Duration:

This stage is typically short-term, lasting until the severe symptoms subside, usually a few days.

Low Fiber Diet:

Purpose:

After the initial flare-up subsides, a low-fiber diet is introduced to transition the digestive system from rest to more normal function. This helps avoid irritation while still providing some nutritional support.

Allowed Foods:

- White bread, refined pasta, and white rice
- Cooked or canned fruits without skins or seeds
- Cooked vegetables without skins or seeds (e.g., carrots, green beans)
- Lean proteins such as poultry, fish, eggs, and tofu
- Dairy products such as milk, yogurt, and cheese (if tolerated)
- Smooth peanut butter and other smooth nut butters

Foods to Avoid:

- Whole grains and high-fiber cereals
- Raw fruits and vegetables
- Nuts, seeds, and popcorn
- Legumes and beans
- Spicy and fatty foods

Duration:

This stage lasts until the digestive system has stabilized and the patient feels ready to reintroduce fiber gradually, usually for a few weeks.

High Fiber Diet:

Purpose:

The high-fiber diet is intended for long-term management of diverticulitis. Adequate fiber intake helps keep the digestive system functioning smoothly by adding bulk to the stool and reducing the pressure on the colon.

Allowed Foods:

- Whole grains such as oatmeal, brown rice, and whole wheat bread
- Fresh fruits such as apples, pears, and berries
- Fresh vegetables such as broccoli, carrots, and spinach
- Legumes and beans (introduced gradually)
- Nuts and seeds (introduced gradually)
- Plenty of water to help fiber digestion

Foods to Avoid:

- Processed and refined foods
- Foods with added sugars and unhealthy fats
- Foods that have previously triggered symptoms

Duration:

This stage is maintained indefinitely as part of a healthy lifestyle to prevent future episodes of diverticulitis.

Foods to Avoid

Avoiding certain foods is crucial in managing diverticulitis, especially during flare-ups and the transition period. These foods can irritate the colon, increase inflammation, and exacerbate symptoms.

During Flare-ups:

High-Fiber Foods:

- Whole grains (brown rice, whole wheat bread)
- Raw fruits and vegetables
- Nuts, seeds, and popcorn
- Legumes and beans

Spicy and Fatty Foods:

- Spicy dishes and sauces
- Fried and greasy foods

Dairy Products:

- Full-fat milk and cheeses (if lactose intolerant)

Caffeinated and Carbonated Beverages:

- Coffee, tea, soda

Alcohol:

- Beer, wine, and spirits

Any food that has previously caused symptoms

Foods to take

Including certain foods in your diet can help manage diverticulitis effectively, promoting healing during flare-ups and supporting long-term digestive health.

During Flare-ups:

Clear Liquids:

- Clear broths (chicken, beef, vegetable)
- Clear juices without pulp (apple, white grape)
- Herbal teas (chamomile, peppermint)
- Gelatin without fruit pieces
- Electrolyte drinks
- Ice pops without fruit or cream

Transition Phase (Low Fiber Diet):

Refined Grains:

- White bread, refined pasta, white rice

Cooked or Canned Fruits:

- Applesauce, canned peaches (without skins or seeds)

Cooked Vegetables:

- Carrots, green beans (without skins or seeds)

Lean Proteins:

- Chicken, turkey, fish, eggs, tofu

Dairy Products:

- Milk, yogurt, cheese (if tolerated)

Smooth Nut Butters:

- Peanut butter (smooth)

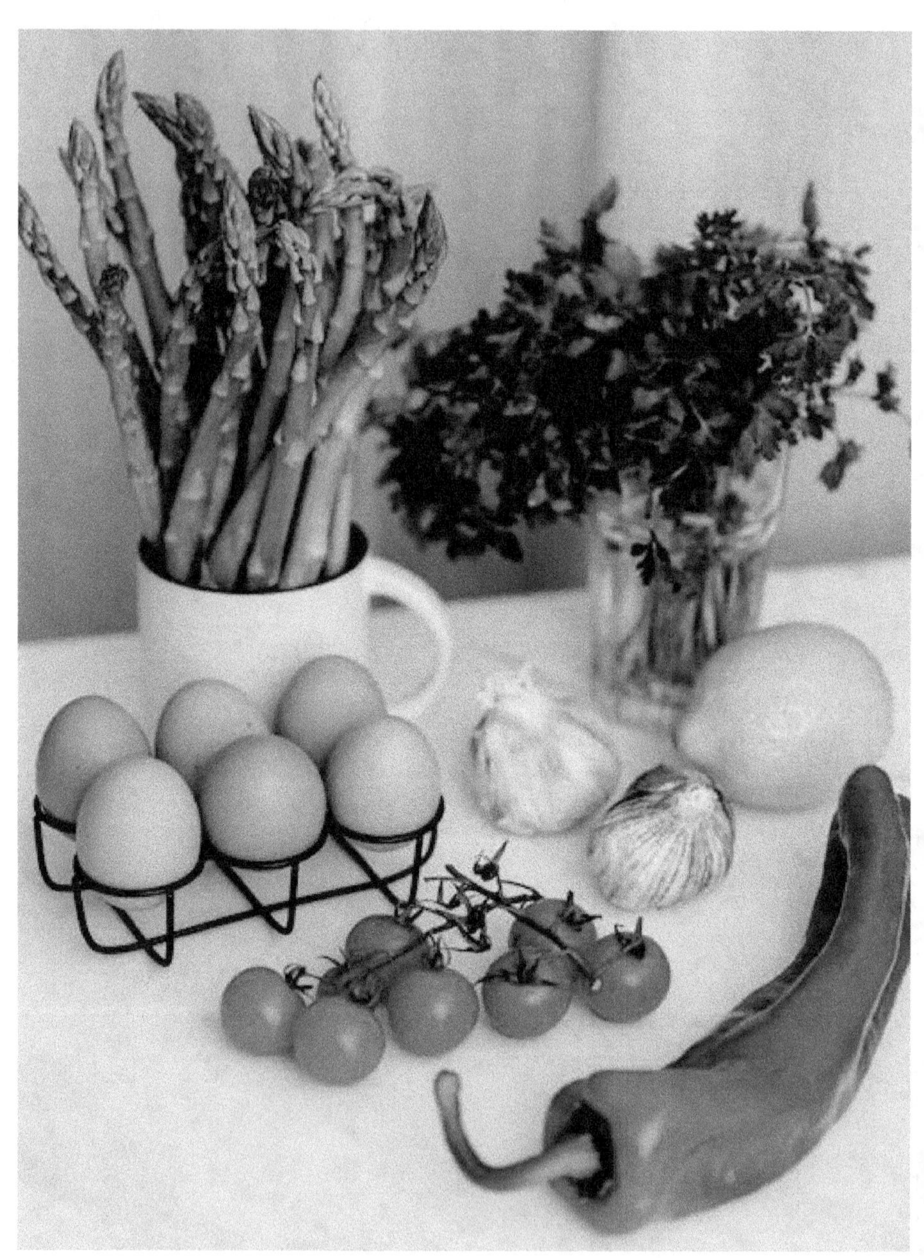

Managing Flare-ups

Managing flare-ups of diverticulitis is crucial to reduce discomfort, promote healing, and prevent complications. A proactive approach involves identifying trigger foods and adjusting the diet appropriately during a flare-up.

Identifying Trigger Foods

Identifying trigger foods is essential for managing diverticulitis flare-ups. These foods can irritate the colon, exacerbate symptoms, and lead to inflammation or infection of the diverticula. Understanding which foods trigger symptoms can help in avoiding them and managing the condition effectively.

Common Trigger Foods:

Nuts and Seeds:

These can get trapped in the diverticula and cause irritation or inflammation. Examples include almonds, sunflower seeds, sesame seeds, and chia seeds.

Popcorn:

The hulls of popcorn can be difficult to digest and may irritate the colon.

Certain Fruits and Vegetables:

Fruits and vegetables with seeds or skins, such as tomatoes, strawberries, raspberries, cucumbers, and bell peppers, can be problematic for some individuals.

Whole Grains:

Foods high in insoluble fiber, such as whole grain bread, brown rice, and bran cereals, can be hard to digest during a flare-up.

Spicy Foods:

Spices and hot peppers can irritate the digestive tract and exacerbate symptoms.

Fatty and Fried Foods:

These can be difficult to digest and may increase the risk of inflammation. Examples include fried chicken, French fries, and fatty cuts of meat.

Dairy Products:

For individuals who are lactose intolerant or sensitive to dairy, products like milk, cheese, and ice cream can cause bloating, gas, and discomfort.

Caffeinated Beverages:

Coffee, tea, and soda can stimulate the digestive tract and worsen symptoms.

Alcohol:

Alcohol can irritate the lining of the colon and lead to inflammation.

Artificial Sweeteners:

Some artificial sweeteners, such as sorbitol and mannitol, can cause digestive upset and bloating.

Methods for Identifying Trigger Foods

Food Diary:

Keep a detailed food diary to track what you eat and any symptoms that follow. Note the type and quantity of food, as well as the timing and severity of symptoms.

Elimination Diet:

Temporarily eliminate suspected trigger foods from your diet and gradually reintroduce them one at a time to identify which foods cause symptoms.

Professional Guidance:

Work with a healthcare provider or dietitian to identify trigger foods and develop a personalized diet plan.

Adjusting the Diet During a Flare-up

During a diverticulitis flare-up, it is important to adjust the diet to minimize discomfort and promote healing. The dietary adjustments typically involve moving through different stages, starting with a clear liquid diet and gradually reintroducing low-fiber foods as symptoms improve.

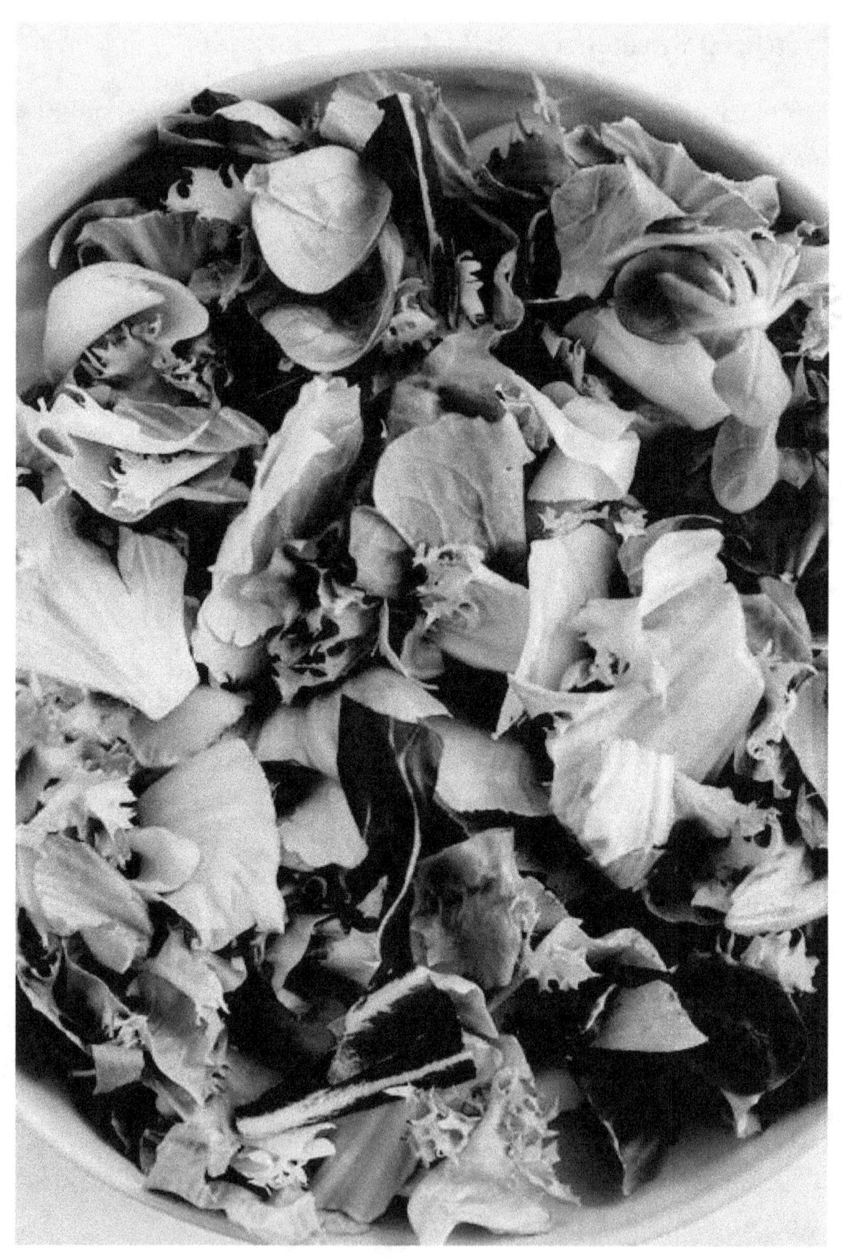

Breakfast Recipes

Oatmeal with Blueberries and Bananas

Ingredients:

- 1 cup rolled oats
- 2 cups water or milk (dairy or plant-based)
- 1/2 cup blueberries
- 1 banana, sliced
- 1 tablespoon honey (optional)

Instructions:

1. In a medium saucepan, bring water or milk to a boil.
2. Add rolled oats, reduce heat to low, and simmer for 5 minutes, stirring occasionally.
3. Remove from heat, cover, and let sit for 2 minutes.
4. Stir in blueberries and sliced banana.
5. Drizzle with honey if desired.

Greek Yogurt with Honey and Soft Fruit

Ingredients:

- 1 cup plain Greek yogurt
- 1 tablespoon honey
- 1/2 cup soft fruit (e.g., ripe bananas, peaches, or pears)

Instructions:

1. Place Greek yogurt in a bowl.
2. Drizzle honey over the yogurt.

3. Top with soft fruit of choice.

Scrambled Eggs with Spinach

Ingredients:

- 2 eggs
- 1/4 cup milk (dairy or plant-based)
- 1/2 cup fresh spinach, chopped
- 1 tablespoon olive oil
- Salt and pepper to taste

Instructions:

1. In a bowl, whisk eggs and milk together until well combined.
2. Heat olive oil in a skillet over medium heat.
3. Add spinach and sauté until wilted, about 2 minutes.
4. Pour in the egg mixture, stirring continuously until eggs are cooked through.
5. Season with salt and pepper to taste.

Smoothie with Banana, Spinach, and Almond Milk

Ingredients:

- 1 banana
- 1 cup fresh spinach
- 1 cup almond milk
- 1 tablespoon almond butter
- 1 tablespoon honey (optional)

Instructions:

1. Place all ingredients in a blender.
2. Blend until smooth.
3. Pour into a glass and enjoy.

Avocado Toast

Ingredients:

- 1 ripe avocado
- 2 slices whole-grain bread
- Salt and pepper to taste

Instructions:

1. Toast the bread slices until golden brown.
2. Mash the avocado in a bowl.
3. Spread the mashed avocado evenly on the toasted bread.
4. Season with salt and pepper.

Cottage Cheese with Peaches

Ingredients:

- 1 cup cottage cheese
- 1 peach, peeled and sliced

Instructions:

1. Place cottage cheese in a bowl.
2. Top with peach slices.

3. Serve immediately.

Quinoa Porridge

Ingredients:

- 1/2 cup quinoa
- 1 cup water
- 1 cup almond milk
- 1 tablespoon honey
- 1/2 teaspoon cinnamon
- 1/4 cup raisins

Instructions:

1. Rinse quinoa under cold water.
2. In a medium saucepan, bring water and quinoa to a boil.
3. Reduce heat, cover, and simmer for 15 minutes or until quinoa is tender.
4. Stir in almond milk, honey, cinnamon, and raisins.
5. Cook for an additional 5 minutes, stirring occasionally.
6. Serve warm.

Chia Pudding with Berries

Ingredients:

- 1/4 cup chia seeds
- 1 cup almond milk
- 1 tablespoon honey

- 1/2 cup mixed berries (e.g., strawberries, blueberries, raspberries)

Instructions:

1. In a bowl, combine chia seeds, almond milk, and honey.
2. Stir well and let sit for 5 minutes.
3. Stir again to prevent clumping.
4. Cover and refrigerate for at least 2 hours or overnight.
5. Top with mixed berries before serving.

Spinach and Feta Omelet

Ingredients:

- 2 eggs
- 1/4 cup milk (dairy or plant-based)
- 1/2 cup fresh spinach, chopped
- 1/4 cup feta cheese, crumbled
- 1 tablespoon olive oil
- Salt and pepper to taste

Instructions:

1. In a bowl, whisk eggs and milk together.
2. Heat olive oil in a skillet over medium heat.
3. Add spinach and sauté until wilted.
4. Pour in the egg mixture and cook until edges start to set.
5. Sprinkle feta cheese over half of the omelet.
6. Fold the omelet in half and cook until fully set.
7. Season with salt and pepper to taste.

Apple and Cinnamon Overnight Oats

Ingredients:

- 1 cup rolled oats
- 1 cup almond milk
- 1 apple, peeled and grated
- 1/2 teaspoon cinnamon
- 1 tablespoon honey

Instructions:

1. In a bowl, combine oats, almond milk, grated apple, cinnamon, and honey.
2. Stir well, cover, and refrigerate overnight.
3. Stir again before serving.

Blueberry Pancakes

Ingredients:

- 1 cup whole wheat flour
- 1 tablespoon baking powder
- 1/2 teaspoon salt
- 1 egg
- 1 cup milk (dairy or plant-based)
- 1 tablespoon honey
- 1 cup blueberries
- Olive oil for cooking

Instructions:

1. In a bowl, combine flour, baking powder, and salt.

2. In another bowl, whisk together egg, milk, and honey.
3. Pour wet ingredients into dry ingredients and mix until just combined.
4. Fold in blueberries.
5. Heat olive oil in a skillet over medium heat.
6. Pour 1/4 cup of batter for each pancake into the skillet.
7. Cook until bubbles form on the surface, then flip and cook until golden brown.
8. Serve warm.

Banana Nut Muffins

Ingredients:

- 2 ripe bananas, mashed
- 1/3 cup olive oil
- 1/2 cup honey
- 2 eggs
- 1/4 cup milk (dairy or plant-based)
- 1 teaspoon vanilla extract
- 1 1/2 cups whole wheat flour
- 1 teaspoon baking soda
- 1/2 teaspoon salt
- 1/2 cup chopped nuts (walnuts or pecans)

Instructions:

1. Preheat oven to 350°F (175°C) and line a muffin tin with paper liners.
2. In a bowl, combine mashed bananas, olive oil, honey, eggs, milk, and vanilla extract.

3. In another bowl, mix flour, baking soda, and salt.
4. Combine wet and dry ingredients until just combined.
5. Fold in chopped nuts.
6. Spoon batter into muffin tin, filling each cup about 2/3 full.
7. Bake for 20-25 minutes or until a toothpick inserted into the center comes out clean.
8. Allow to cool before serving.

Smoothie Bowl with Mixed Berries

Ingredients:

- 1 banana
- 1/2 cup mixed berries (e.g., strawberries, blueberries, raspberries)
- 1/2 cup Greek yogurt
- 1/2 cup almond milk
- 1 tablespoon honey
- Toppings: granola, chia seeds, fresh berries

Instructions:

1. Blend banana, mixed berries, Greek yogurt, almond milk, and honey until smooth.
2. Pour into a bowl.
3. Top with granola, chia seeds, and fresh berries.

Poached Eggs with Avocado

Ingredients:

- 2 eggs
- 1 ripe avocado
- 2 slices whole-grain bread
- 1 tablespoon olive oil
- Salt and pepper to taste

Instructions:

1. Bring a pot of water to a gentle simmer.
2. Crack eggs into separate small bowls.
3. Carefully slide eggs into simmering water and poach for 3-4 minutes until whites are set.
4. Toast the bread slices.
5. Mash the avocado and spread evenly on toasted bread.
6. Top each slice with a poached egg.
7. Drizzle with olive oil and season with salt and pepper.

Millet Porridge with Apple and Cinnamon

Ingredients:

- 1/2 cup millet
- 1 cup water
- 1 cup almond milk
- 1 apple, peeled and diced
- 1/2 teaspoon cinnamon
- 1 tablespoon honey

Instructions:

1. Rinse millet under cold water.
2. In a medium saucepan, bring water and millet to a boil.

3. Reduce heat, cover, and simmer for 20 minutes.
4. Stir in almond milk, diced apple, cinnamon, and honey.
5. Cook for an additional 5-10 minutes, stirring occasionally.
6. Serve warm.

Soft-Boiled Eggs with Whole-Grain Toast

Ingredients:

- 2 eggs
- 2 slices whole-grain bread
- 1 tablespoon butter
- Salt and pepper to taste

Instructions:

1. Bring a pot of water to a gentle boil.
2. Lower eggs into the water and boil for 6 minutes.
3. Toast the bread slices and spread with butter.
4. Remove eggs from water and place in ice water for 1 minute.
5. Peel eggs and serve with buttered toast.
6. Season with salt and pepper.

Buckwheat Pancakes

Ingredients:

- 1 cup buckwheat flour
- 1 tablespoon baking powder
- 1/2 teaspoon salt

- 1 egg
- 1 cup almond milk
- 1 tablespoon honey
- Olive oil for cooking

Instructions:

1. In a bowl, combine buckwheat flour, baking powder, and salt.
2. In another bowl, whisk together egg, almond milk, and honey.
3. Pour wet ingredients into dry ingredients and mix until just combined.
4. Heat olive oil in a skillet over medium heat.
5. Pour 1/4 cup of batter for each pancake into the skillet.
6. Cook until bubbles form on the surface, then flip and cook until golden brown.
7. Serve warm.

Cottage Cheese Pancakes

Ingredients:

- 1 cup cottage cheese
- 2 eggs
- 1/4 cup whole wheat flour
- 1/2 teaspoon baking powder
- 1 tablespoon honey
- Olive oil for cooking

Instructions:

1. In a bowl, combine cottage cheese, eggs, flour, baking powder, and honey.
2. Mix until well combined.
3. Heat olive oil in a skillet over medium heat.
4. Pour 1/4 cup of batter for each pancake into the skillet.
5. Cook until bubbles form on the surface, then flip and cook until golden brown.
6. Serve warm.

Berry and Yogurt Parfait

Ingredients:

- 1 cup plain Greek yogurt
- 1/2 cup mixed berries (e.g., strawberries, blueberries, raspberries)
- 1/4 cup granola
- 1 tablespoon honey

Instructions:

1. In a glass or bowl, layer half of the yogurt, berries, granola, and honey.
2. Repeat the layers with the remaining yogurt, berries, granola, and honey.
3. Serve immediately.

Baked Apple with Cinnamon

Ingredients:

- 1 apple, cored
- 1 tablespoon honey
- 1/2 teaspoon cinnamon
- 1 tablespoon raisins
- 1 tablespoon chopped nuts (optional)

Instructions:

1. Preheat oven to 350°F (175°C).
2. Place the cored apple in a baking dish.
3. Fill the center of the apple with honey, cinnamon, raisins, and nuts if using.
4. Bake for 25-30 minutes or until the apple is tender.
5. Serve warm.

Lunch Recipes

Chicken and Vegetable Soup

Ingredients:

- 1 boneless, skinless chicken breast, diced
- 4 cups low-sodium chicken broth
- 1 cup carrots, diced
- 1 cup green beans, chopped
- 1 cup potatoes, diced
- 1 tablespoon olive oil
- Salt and pepper to taste

Instructions:

1. Heat olive oil in a large pot over medium heat.
2. Add diced chicken and cook until no longer pink.
3. Add chicken broth, carrots, green beans, and potatoes.
4. Bring to a boil, then reduce heat and simmer for 20 minutes or until vegetables are tender.
5. Season with salt and pepper to taste. Serve warm.

Turkey and Avocado Wrap

Ingredients:

- 1 whole-grain tortilla
- 3 slices turkey breast
- 1/2 avocado, sliced
- 1/4 cup shredded lettuce
- 1 tablespoon low-fat mayonnaise

Instructions:

1. Spread mayonnaise evenly over the tortilla.
2. Layer turkey slices, avocado, and lettuce.
3. Roll up the tortilla tightly and slice in half. Serve immediately.

Quinoa Salad with Cucumber and Feta

Ingredients:

- 1 cup cooked quinoa
- 1/2 cup cucumber, diced
- 1/4 cup crumbled feta cheese
- 2 tablespoons olive oil
- 1 tablespoon lemon juice
- Salt and pepper to taste

Instructions:

1. In a bowl, combine cooked quinoa, cucumber, and feta cheese.
2. In a small bowl, whisk together olive oil and lemon juice.
3. Pour dressing over the quinoa mixture and toss to combine.
4. Season with salt and pepper to taste. Serve chilled or at room temperature.

Baked Sweet Potato with Greek Yogurt

Ingredients:

- 1 large sweet potato
- 1/2 cup plain Greek yogurt
- 1 tablespoon honey
- 1/4 teaspoon cinnamon

Instructions:

1. Preheat oven to 400°F (200°C).
2. Pierce the sweet potato with a fork and bake for 45-60 minutes or until tender.
3. Cut open the sweet potato and top with Greek yogurt, honey, and cinnamon.
4. Serve warm.

Lentil Soup

Ingredients:

- 1 cup lentils, rinsed
- 4 cups vegetable broth
- 1 cup carrots, diced
- 1 cup celery, diced
- 1 tablespoon olive oil
- 1 teaspoon dried thyme
- Salt and pepper to taste

Instructions:

1. Heat olive oil in a large pot over medium heat.
2. Add carrots and celery, cooking until softened.
3. Add lentils, vegetable broth, and thyme.

4. Bring to a boil, then reduce heat and simmer for 30 minutes or until lentils are tender.
5. Season with salt and pepper to taste. Serve warm.

Spinach and Egg Salad

Ingredients:

- 2 hard-boiled eggs, chopped
- 2 cups fresh spinach
- 1/4 cup cherry tomatoes, halved
- 1 tablespoon olive oil
- 1 tablespoon balsamic vinegar
- Salt and pepper to taste

Instructions:

1. In a large bowl, combine spinach, cherry tomatoes, and chopped eggs.
2. In a small bowl, whisk together olive oil and balsamic vinegar.
3. Drizzle dressing over the salad and toss to combine.
4. Season with salt and pepper to taste. Serve immediately.

Stuffed Bell Peppers

Ingredients:

- 4 bell peppers, tops cut off and seeds removed
- 1 cup cooked brown rice
- 1 cup ground turkey, cooked

- 1/2 cup tomato sauce
- 1/4 cup shredded mozzarella cheese
- 1 tablespoon olive oil
- Salt and pepper to taste

Instructions:

1. Preheat oven to 375°F (190°C).
2. In a bowl, mix cooked rice, ground turkey, tomato sauce, and half of the cheese.
3. Stuff each bell pepper with the mixture.
4. Place stuffed peppers in a baking dish, drizzle with olive oil, and sprinkle with remaining cheese.
5. Bake for 25-30 minutes or until peppers are tender. Serve warm.

Chicken and Apple Salad

Ingredients:

- 1 cooked chicken breast, diced
- 1 apple, diced
- 1/4 cup celery, diced
- 2 tablespoons plain Greek yogurt
- 1 tablespoon honey
- Salt and pepper to taste

Instructions:

1. In a bowl, combine chicken, apple, and celery.
2. In a small bowl, mix Greek yogurt and honey.
3. Add dressing to the chicken mixture and toss to combine.

4. Season with salt and pepper to taste. Serve chilled.

Creamy Butternut Squash Soup

Ingredients:

- 1 butternut squash, peeled and cubed
- 4 cups vegetable broth
- 1 onion, diced
- 1 tablespoon olive oil
- 1/2 cup plain Greek yogurt
- Salt and pepper to taste

Instructions:

1. Heat olive oil in a large pot over medium heat.
2. Add onion and cook until softened.
3. Add butternut squash and vegetable broth. Bring to a boil, then reduce heat and simmer for 20 minutes or until squash is tender.
4. Puree the soup with an immersion blender or in batches in a blender.
5. Stir in Greek yogurt and season with salt and pepper. Serve warm.

Turkey and Spinach Stuffed Mushrooms

Ingredients:

- 12 large mushrooms, stems removed
- 1 cup cooked ground turkey

- 1/2 cup fresh spinach, chopped
- 1/4 cup breadcrumbs
- 1/4 cup grated Parmesan cheese
- 1 tablespoon olive oil
- Salt and pepper to taste

Instructions:

1. Preheat oven to 375°F (190°C).
2. In a bowl, combine ground turkey, spinach, breadcrumbs, and Parmesan cheese.
3. Stuff each mushroom cap with the turkey mixture.
4. Place stuffed mushrooms in a baking dish, drizzle with olive oil, and bake for 20 minutes or until mushrooms are tender. Serve warm.

Zucchini Noodles with Tomato Sauce

Ingredients:

- 2 large zucchinis, spiralized into noodles
- 1 cup tomato sauce
- 1 tablespoon olive oil
- 1/4 cup grated Parmesan cheese
- Salt and pepper to taste

Instructions:

1. Heat olive oil in a skillet over medium heat.
2. Add zucchini noodles and cook for 3-4 minutes until tender.
3. Stir in tomato sauce and cook until heated through.

4. Season with salt and pepper.
5. Sprinkle with Parmesan cheese before serving.

Eggplant and Tomato Bake

Ingredients:

- 1 large eggplant, sliced
- 2 cups tomato sauce
- 1/2 cup shredded mozzarella cheese
- 1 tablespoon olive oil
- 1/2 teaspoon dried basil
- Salt and pepper to taste

Instructions:

1. Preheat oven to 375°F (190°C).
2. Brush eggplant slices with olive oil and place on a baking sheet.
3. Bake for 20 minutes, flipping halfway through.
4. In a baking dish, layer baked eggplant slices with tomato sauce and mozzarella cheese.
5. Bake for an additional 15 minutes or until cheese is melted. Serve warm.

Salmon with Steamed Broccoli

Ingredients:

- 2 salmon fillets
- 1 tablespoon olive oil

- 1 lemon, sliced
- 1 cup broccoli florets
- Salt and pepper to taste

Instructions:

1. Preheat oven to 375°F (190°C).
2. Place salmon fillets on a baking sheet, drizzle with olive oil, and season with salt and pepper.
3. Top with lemon slices and bake for 15-20 minutes or until salmon is cooked through.
4. Steam broccoli until tender, about 5 minutes.
5. Serve salmon with steamed broccoli.

Chicken and Quinoa Stuffed Bell Peppers

Ingredients:

- 4 bell peppers, tops cut off and seeds removed
- 1 cup cooked quinoa
- 1 cup cooked chicken breast, diced
- 1/2 cup tomato sauce
- 1/4 cup shredded cheddar cheese
- 1 tablespoon olive oil
- Salt and pepper to taste

Instructions:

1. Preheat oven to 375°F (190°C).
2. In a bowl, mix quinoa, chicken, tomato sauce, and half of the cheese.
3. Stuff each bell pepper with the mixture.

4. Place stuffed peppers in a baking dish, drizzle with olive oil, and sprinkle with remaining cheese.
5. Bake for 25-30 minutes or until peppers are tender. Serve warm.

Roasted Vegetable and Hummus Wrap

Ingredients:

- 1 whole-grain tortilla
- 1/2 cup roasted vegetables (e.g., zucchini, bell peppers, carrots)
- 2 tablespoons hummus
- 1/4 cup fresh spinach

Instructions:

1. Spread hummus evenly over the tortilla.
2. Layer with roasted vegetables and fresh spinach.
3. Roll up the tortilla tightly and slice in half. Serve immediately.

Cauliflower Rice Stir-Fry

Ingredients:

- 2 cups cauliflower rice
- 1 cup mixed vegetables (e.g., peas, carrots, bell peppers)
- 1 tablespoon olive oil
- 2 tablespoons low-sodium soy sauce
- 1/2 teaspoon garlic powder

Instructions:

1. Heat olive oil in a skillet over medium heat.
2. Add mixed vegetables and cook until tender.
3. Stir in cauliflower rice and cook for 5-7 minutes.
4. Add soy sauce and garlic powder, stirring to combine.
5. Serve warm.

Tuna Salad Lettuce Wraps

Ingredients:

- 1 can tuna, drained
- 1/4 cup plain Greek yogurt
- 1 tablespoon Dijon mustard
- 1/4 cup diced celery
- 1/4 cup diced red pepper
- Large lettuce leaves

Instructions:

1. In a bowl, combine tuna, Greek yogurt, Dijon mustard, celery, and red pepper.
2. Spoon the mixture onto lettuce leaves.
3. Wrap and serve immediately.

Chicken and Avocado Salad

Ingredients:

- 1 cooked chicken breast, diced

- 1 avocado, diced
- 1/4 cup diced red onion
- 2 cups mixed greens
- 2 tablespoons olive oil
- 1 tablespoon lemon juice
- Salt and pepper to taste

Instructions:

1. In a large bowl, combine chicken, avocado, red onion, and mixed greens.
2. In a small bowl, whisk together olive oil and lemon juice.
3. Drizzle dressing over the salad and toss to combine.
4. Season with salt and pepper to taste. Serve immediately.

Sweet Potato and Black Bean Bowl

Ingredients:

- 1 large sweet potato, peeled and diced
- 1 cup black beans, drained and rinsed
- 1/2 cup corn kernels
- 1 tablespoon olive oil
- 1/2 teaspoon cumin
- Salt and pepper to taste

Instructions:

1. Preheat oven to 400°F (200°C).
2. Toss sweet potato with olive oil, cumin, salt, and pepper.
3. Spread on a baking sheet and roast for 25-30 minutes or until tender.

4. In a bowl, combine roasted sweet potato, black beans, and corn.
5. Serve warm.

Creamy Spinach and Mushroom Quiche

Ingredients:

- 1 whole-grain pie crust
- 1 cup fresh spinach, chopped
- 1/2 cup mushrooms, sliced
- 3 eggs
- 1 cup milk (dairy or plant-based)
- 1/4 cup shredded cheese (e.g., cheddar or mozzarella)
- Salt and pepper to taste

Instructions:

1. Preheat oven to 375°F (190°C).
2. In a skillet, sauté mushrooms until tender. Add spinach and cook until wilted.
3. In a bowl, whisk together eggs and milk.
4. Stir in the mushroom and spinach mixture, and cheese.
5. Pour into the pie crust and bake for 35-40 minutes or until set.
6. Allow to cool slightly before slicing. Serve warm.

These recipes offer a range of options that are gentle on the digestive system and suitable for managing diverticulitis. Adjust seasonings and ingredients based on your tolerance and preferences.

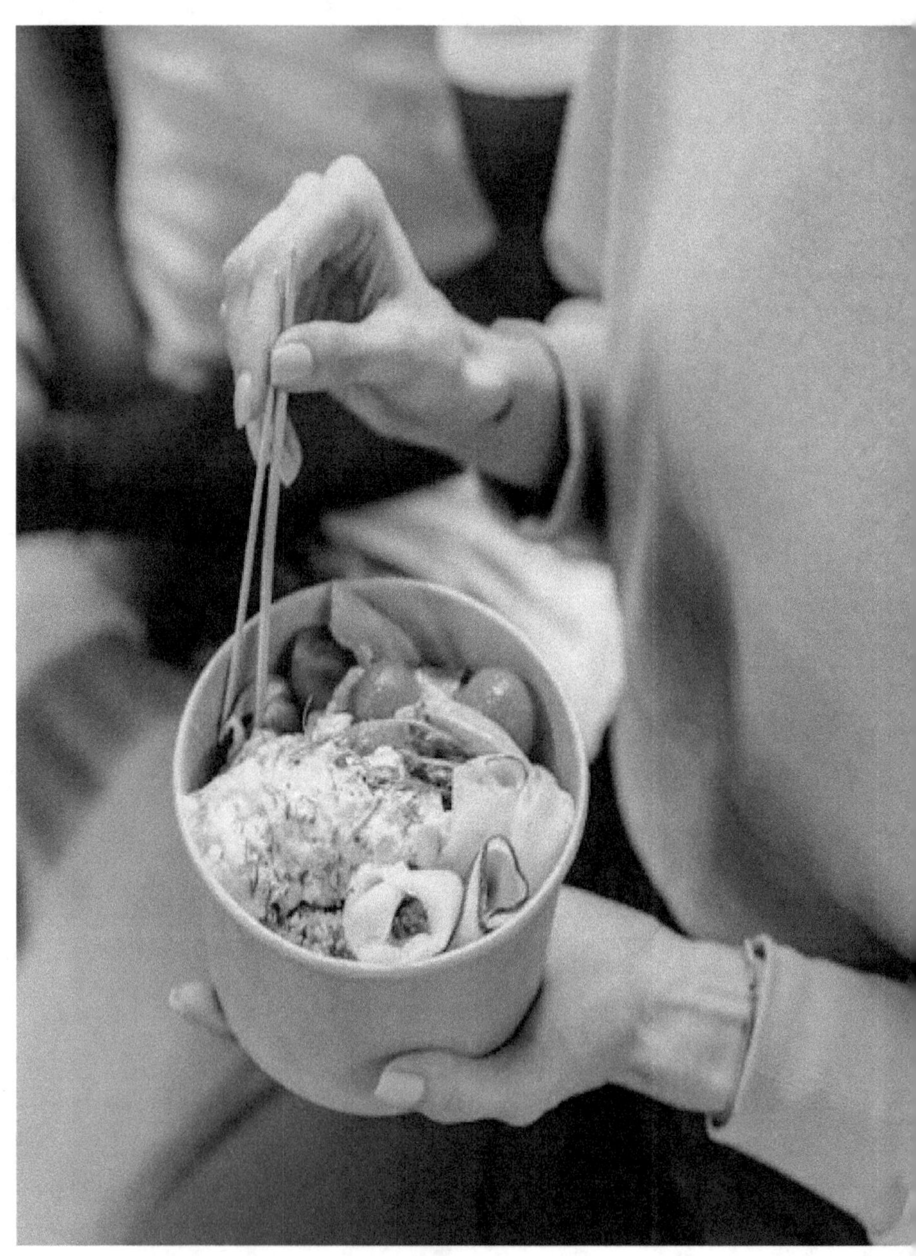

Dinner Recipes

Baked Salmon with Asparagus

Ingredients:

- 2 salmon fillets
- 1 bunch asparagus, trimmed
- 2 tablespoons olive oil
- 1 lemon, sliced
- Salt and pepper to taste

Instructions:

1. Preheat oven to 400°F (200°C).
2. Place salmon fillets and asparagus on a baking sheet.
3. Drizzle with olive oil and season with salt and pepper.
4. Top salmon with lemon slices.
5. Bake for 15-20 minutes or until salmon is cooked through and asparagus is tender. Serve warm.

Chicken and Sweet Potato Bake

Ingredients:

- 2 boneless, skinless chicken breasts
- 2 large sweet potatoes, peeled and diced
- 2 tablespoons olive oil
- 1 teaspoon dried rosemary
- Salt and pepper to taste

Instructions:

1. Preheat oven to 375°F (190°C).
2. Toss sweet potatoes with olive oil, rosemary, salt, and pepper.
3. Place sweet potatoes in a baking dish and top with chicken breasts.
4. Bake for 30-35 minutes or until chicken is cooked through and sweet potatoes are tender. Serve warm.

Turkey and Spinach Stuffed Zucchini

Ingredients:

- 4 medium zucchinis, halved lengthwise
- 1 cup ground turkey
- 1 cup fresh spinach, chopped
- 1/2 cup tomato sauce
- 1/4 cup shredded mozzarella cheese
- 1 tablespoon olive oil
- Salt and pepper to taste

Instructions:

1. Preheat oven to 375°F (190°C).
2. Heat olive oil in a skillet over medium heat. Cook ground turkey until browned.
3. Stir in spinach and cook until wilted.
4. Fill zucchini halves with the turkey mixture.
5. Top with tomato sauce and cheese.
6. Place in a baking dish and bake for 20-25 minutes or until zucchini is tender. Serve warm.

Lentil and Vegetable Stew

Ingredients:

- 1 cup lentils, rinsed
- 4 cups vegetable broth
- 1 cup carrots, diced
- 1 cup celery, diced
- 1 cup potatoes, diced
- 1 tablespoon olive oil
- 1 teaspoon dried thyme
- Salt and pepper to taste

Instructions:

1. Heat olive oil in a large pot over medium heat.
2. Add carrots, celery, and potatoes; cook until slightly softened.
3. Stir in lentils, vegetable broth, and thyme.
4. Bring to a boil, then reduce heat and simmer for 30 minutes or until lentils and vegetables are tender.
5. Season with salt and pepper. Serve warm.

Baked Chicken with Carrots and Parsnips

Ingredients:

- 2 boneless, skinless chicken thighs
- 2 large carrots, peeled and sliced
- 2 parsnips, peeled and sliced
- 2 tablespoons olive oil
- 1 teaspoon dried thyme

- Salt and pepper to taste

Instructions:

1. Preheat oven to 375°F (190°C).
2. Toss carrots and parsnips with olive oil, thyme, salt, and pepper.
3. Place in a baking dish and top with chicken thighs.
4. Bake for 30-35 minutes or until chicken is cooked through and vegetables are tender. Serve warm.

Quinoa-Stuffed Bell Peppers

Ingredients:

- 4 bell peppers, tops cut off and seeds removed
- 1 cup cooked quinoa
- 1 cup diced tomatoes
- 1/2 cup black beans, rinsed
- 1/4 cup shredded cheese (optional)
- 1 tablespoon olive oil
- Salt and pepper to taste

Instructions:

1. Preheat oven to 375°F (190°C).
2. In a bowl, mix quinoa, diced tomatoes, black beans, and half of the cheese.
3. Stuff bell peppers with the quinoa mixture.
4. Place in a baking dish, drizzle with olive oil, and top with remaining cheese.

5. Bake for 25-30 minutes or until peppers are tender. Serve warm.

Creamy Cauliflower Soup

Ingredients:

- 1 large cauliflower, chopped
- 4 cups vegetable broth
- 1 onion, diced
- 2 tablespoons olive oil
- 1/2 cup plain Greek yogurt
- Salt and pepper to taste

Instructions:

1. Heat olive oil in a large pot over medium heat. Cook onion until softened.
2. Add cauliflower and vegetable broth. Bring to a boil, then reduce heat and simmer for 20 minutes or until cauliflower is tender.
3. Puree the soup with an immersion blender or in batches in a blender.
4. Stir in Greek yogurt and season with salt and pepper. Serve warm.

Turkey Meatballs with Steamed Broccoli

Ingredients:

- 1 lb ground turkey

- 1/4 cup breadcrumbs
- 1 egg
- 1/4 cup grated Parmesan cheese
- 1 teaspoon dried oregano
- 1/4 teaspoon garlic powder
- 1 cup broccoli florets

Instructions:

1. Preheat oven to 375°F (190°C).
2. In a bowl, mix ground turkey, breadcrumbs, egg, Parmesan cheese, oregano, and garlic powder.
3. Form mixture into meatballs and place on a baking sheet.
4. Bake for 20-25 minutes or until cooked through.
5. Steam broccoli until tender, about 5 minutes.
6. Serve meatballs with steamed broccoli.

Baked Cod with Spinach

Ingredients:

- 2 cod fillets
- 2 cups fresh spinach
- 2 tablespoons olive oil
- 1 lemon, sliced
- Salt and pepper to taste

Instructions:

1. Preheat oven to 400°F (200°C).
2. Place cod fillets on a baking sheet and drizzle with olive oil.

3. Top with lemon slices and season with salt and pepper.
4. Bake for 15-20 minutes or until cod is cooked through.
5. Serve with fresh spinach.

Chicken and Broccoli Stir-Fry

Ingredients:

- 2 boneless, skinless chicken breasts, sliced
- 2 cups broccoli florets
- 1 tablespoon olive oil
- 2 tablespoons low-sodium soy sauce
- 1/2 teaspoon ginger powder

Instructions:

1. Heat olive oil in a skillet over medium heat.
2. Add chicken and cook until browned.
3. Add broccoli and cook until tender-crisp.
4. Stir in soy sauce and ginger powder.
5. Cook for an additional 2-3 minutes. Serve warm.

Spaghetti Squash with Tomato Sauce

Ingredients:

- 1 medium spaghetti squash
- 1 cup tomato sauce
- 1/4 cup grated Parmesan cheese
- 1 tablespoon olive oil
- Salt and pepper to taste

Instructions:

1. Preheat oven to 400°F (200°C).
2. Cut spaghetti squash in half and scoop out seeds.
3. Brush with olive oil, season with salt and pepper, and place cut-side down on a baking sheet.
4. Bake for 40-45 minutes or until tender.
5. Use a fork to scrape the squash into strands. Top with tomato sauce and Parmesan cheese. Serve warm.

Eggplant Parmesan

Ingredients:

- 1 large eggplant, sliced
- 1 cup tomato sauce
- 1/2 cup shredded mozzarella cheese
- 1/4 cup grated Parmesan cheese
- 1/2 cup whole wheat breadcrumbs
- 2 tablespoons olive oil
- Salt and pepper to taste

Instructions:

1. Preheat oven to 375°F (190°C).
2. Brush eggplant slices with olive oil and place on a baking sheet.
3. Bake for 20 minutes, flipping halfway through.
4. In a baking dish, layer eggplant slices with tomato sauce, mozzarella, and Parmesan cheese.
5. Sprinkle with breadcrumbs and bake for an additional 15 minutes or until cheese is melted. Serve warm.

Baked Chicken and Green Beans

Ingredients:

- 2 boneless, skinless chicken breasts
- 2 cups green beans, trimmed
- 2 tablespoons olive oil
- 1 teaspoon dried thyme
- Salt and pepper to taste

Instructions:

1. Preheat oven to 375°F (190°C).
2. Toss green beans with olive oil, thyme, salt, and pepper.
3. Place green beans in a baking dish and top with chicken breasts.
4. Bake for 25-30 minutes or until chicken is cooked through and green beans are tender. Serve warm.

Stuffed Acorn Squash

Ingredients:

- 2 acorn squash, halved and seeded
- 1 cup cooked wild rice
- 1/2 cup dried cranberries
- 1/4 cup chopped walnuts
- 1 tablespoon olive oil
- Salt and pepper to taste

Instructions:

1. Preheat oven to 375°F (190°C).

2. Brush squash with olive oil and season with salt and pepper.
3. Place cut-side down on a baking sheet and bake for 30 minutes.
4. In a bowl, combine cooked rice, cranberries, and walnuts.
5. Turn squash cut-side up and fill with the rice mixture.
6. Bake for an additional 10-15 minutes. Serve warm.

Chicken and Vegetable Stir-Fry

Ingredients:

- 2 boneless, skinless chicken breasts, sliced
- 1 cup snap peas
- 1 cup bell peppers, sliced
- 1 tablespoon olive oil
- 2 tablespoons low-sodium soy sauce
- 1/2 teaspoon ginger powder

Instructions:

1. Heat olive oil in a skillet over medium heat.
2. Add chicken and cook until browned.
3. Add snap peas and bell peppers and stir-fry until tender.
4. Stir in soy sauce and ginger powder.
5. Cook for an additional 2-3 minutes. Serve warm.

Sweet Potato and Black Bean Chili

Ingredients:

- 1 large sweet potato, peeled and diced
- 1 cup black beans, drained and rinsed
- 1 cup diced tomatoes
- 1 tablespoon olive oil
- 1 teaspoon chili powder
- Salt and pepper to taste

Instructions:

1. Heat olive oil in a large pot over medium heat.
2. Add sweet potato and cook for 5 minutes.
3. Stir in black beans, tomatoes, chili powder, salt, and pepper.
4. Simmer for 20-25 minutes or until sweet potato is tender. Serve warm.

Cod and Vegetable Foil Packets

Ingredients:

- 2 cod fillets
- 1 cup baby potatoes, halved
- 1 cup bell peppers, sliced
- 1 tablespoon olive oil
- 1 lemon, sliced
- Salt and pepper to taste

Instructions:

1. Preheat oven to 400°F (200°C).
2. Cut two large pieces of aluminum foil and place cod fillets in the center.

3. Top with potatoes, bell peppers, lemon slices, and drizzle with olive oil.
4. Fold foil into packets and bake for 20-25 minutes or until cod is cooked through and vegetables are tender. Serve warm.

Chicken and Avocado Salad

Ingredients:

- 1 cooked chicken breast, diced
- 1 avocado, diced
- 1/4 cup cherry tomatoes, halved
- 2 cups mixed greens
- 2 tablespoons olive oil
- 1 tablespoon lemon juice
- Salt and pepper to taste

Instructions:

1. In a large bowl, combine chicken, avocado, cherry tomatoes, and mixed greens.
2. In a small bowl, whisk together olive oil and lemon juice.
3. Drizzle dressing over the salad and toss to combine.
4. Season with salt and pepper to taste. Serve immediately.

Stuffed Portobello Mushrooms

Ingredients:

- 4 large portobello mushrooms, stems removed

- 1 cup cooked quinoa
- 1/2 cup diced tomatoes
- 1/4 cup shredded mozzarella cheese
- 1 tablespoon olive oil
- Salt and pepper to taste

Instructions:

1. Preheat oven to 375°F (190°C).
2. In a bowl, mix quinoa, diced tomatoes, and half of the cheese.
3. Stuff each mushroom cap with the mixture.
4. Place in a baking dish, drizzle with olive oil, and top with remaining cheese.
5. Bake for 20 minutes or until mushrooms are tender. Serve warm.

Spinach and Mushroom Frittata

Ingredients:

- 6 eggs
- 1 cup fresh spinach, chopped
- 1/2 cup mushrooms, sliced
- 1/4 cup milk (dairy or plant-based)
- 1/4 cup shredded cheese (e.g., cheddar or mozzarella)
- 1 tablespoon olive oil
- Salt and pepper to taste

Instructions:

1. Preheat oven to 375°F (190°C).

2. Heat olive oil in an oven-safe skillet over medium heat. Cook mushrooms until tender.
3. Add spinach and cook until wilted.
4. In a bowl, whisk together eggs, milk, cheese, salt, and pepper.
5. Pour egg mixture over vegetables in the skillet.
6. Transfer skillet to the oven and bake for 20-25 minutes or until set. Serve warm.

21 Days Meal Plan

Day 1

Breakfast: Chicken and Vegetable Soup

Lunch: Turkey and Avocado Wrap

Dinner: Baked Salmon with Asparagus

Day 2

Breakfast: Quinoa Salad with Cucumber and Feta

Lunch: Spinach and Egg Salad

Dinner: Turkey and Spinach Stuffed Zucchini

Day 3

Breakfast: Baked Sweet Potato with Greek Yogurt

Lunch: Stuffed Bell Peppers

Dinner: Lentil and Vegetable Stew

Day 4

Breakfast: Spinach and Egg Salad

Lunch: Chicken and Apple Salad

Dinner: Baked Chicken with Carrots and Parsnips

Day 5

Breakfast: Creamy Butternut Squash Soup

Lunch: Roasted Vegetable and Hummus Wrap

Dinner: Quinoa-Stuffed Bell Peppers

Day 6

Breakfast: Turkey and Avocado Wrap

Lunch: Chicken and Quinoa Stuffed Bell Peppers

Dinner: Baked Cod with Spinach

Day 7

Breakfast: Creamy Butternut Squash Soup

Lunch: Tuna Salad Lettuce Wraps

Dinner: Chicken and Broccoli Stir-Fry

Day 8

Breakfast: Chicken and Vegetable Soup

Lunch: Chicken and Apple Salad

Dinner: Eggplant Parmesan

Day 9

Breakfast: Quinoa Salad with Cucumber and Feta

Lunch: Spinach and Egg Salad

Dinner: Sweet Potato and Black Bean Chili

Day 10

Breakfast: Baked Sweet Potato with Greek Yogurt

Lunch: Stuffed Acorn Squash

Dinner: Baked Chicken and Green Beans

Day 11

Breakfast: Creamy Butternut Squash Soup

Lunch: Roasted Vegetable and Hummus Wrap

Dinner: Cod and Vegetable Foil Packets

Day 12

Breakfast: Turkey and Avocado Wrap

Lunch: Chicken and Quinoa Stuffed Bell Peppers

Dinner: Stuffed Portobello Mushrooms

Day 13

Breakfast: Spinach and Egg Salad

Lunch: Tuna Salad Lettuce Wraps

Dinner: Spinach and Mushroom Frittata

Day 14

Breakfast: Baked Sweet Potato with Greek Yogurt

Lunch: Turkey and Spinach Stuffed Zucchini

Dinner: Chicken and Sweet Potato Bake

Day 15

Breakfast: Creamy Butternut Squash Soup

Lunch: Chicken and Apple Salad

Dinner: Spaghetti Squash with Tomato Sauce

Day 16

Breakfast: Quinoa Salad with Cucumber and Feta

Lunch: Roasted Vegetable and Hummus Wrap

Dinner: Sweet Potato and Black Bean Bowl

Day 17

Breakfast: Chicken and Vegetable Soup

Lunch: Spinach and Egg Salad

Dinner: Turkey Meatballs with Steamed Broccoli

Day 18

Breakfast: Baked Sweet Potato with Greek Yogurt

Lunch: Stuffed Acorn Squash

Dinner: Chicken and Avocado Salad

Day 19

Breakfast: Creamy Butternut Squash Soup

Lunch: Chicken and Quinoa Stuffed Bell Peppers

Dinner: Eggplant Parmesan

Day 20

Breakfast: Quinoa Salad with Cucumber and Feta

Lunch: Roasted Vegetable and Hummus Wrap

Dinner: Chicken and Broccoli Stir-Fry

Day 21

Breakfast: Chicken and Vegetable Soup

Lunch: Tuna Salad Lettuce Wraps

Dinner: Spinach and Mushroom Frittata

This meal plan offers a variety of nutrient-dense and easy-to-digest options, making it easier to manage diverticulitis while ensuring balanced nutrition. Feel free to adjust portions or ingredients based on your preferences and tolerance.

Conclusion

Navigating a diet tailored for diverticulitis can be challenging, but with the right guidance and resources, it becomes manageable and even enjoyable. This cookbook has been crafted to provide a comprehensive approach to meal planning that accommodates the dietary needs of those with diverticulitis while ensuring meals remain flavorful and satisfying.

A carefully managed diet is crucial for those with diverticulitis to help manage symptoms, prevent flare-ups, and promote overall digestive health. Understanding what foods are beneficial and which ones to avoid can make a significant difference in maintaining comfort and well-being. This cookbook offers a variety of recipes designed to be gentle on the digestive system while providing essential nutrients and flavors.

The recipes included in this cookbook emphasize the importance of:

- Low-FODMAP Ingredients: To minimize digestive discomfort, many recipes focus on low-FODMAP ingredients that are less likely to trigger symptoms.
- Fiber Management: Balancing fiber intake is crucial. The recipes are designed to include sources of soluble fiber, which can help soothe the digestive tract and promote regularity without causing irritation.
- Avoiding Common Triggers: Ingredients that can exacerbate symptoms, such as high-fat, spicy, or overly processed foods, are consciously omitted or substituted with more suitable alternatives.

The 21-day meal plan provided incorporates a diverse array of recipes, ensuring variety and balanced nutrition while adhering to dietary restrictions. From breakfasts that start the day right to lunches that are both filling and easy on the digestive system, and dinners that are both comforting and nutritious, the plan covers all the bases. Each meal has been selected to provide essential nutrients, support digestive health, and offer a range of flavors to keep meals enjoyable.

Adhering to a diverticulitis-friendly diet doesn't mean sacrificing flavor or satisfaction. With the right recipes and a bit of creativity, meals can be both healthful and delicious. This cookbook aims to make meal planning easier and more enjoyable, providing a resource that supports both dietary needs and culinary pleasure.

While the provided recipes and meal plan serve as a solid foundation, it is important to remember that individual needs and tolerances may vary. Personalizing the meal plan based on specific dietary reactions, preferences, and nutritional requirements will enhance the overall experience. Adjusting recipes and experimenting with different ingredients within the guidelines of a diverticulitis diet can help in finding what works best for you.

As you move forward with your dietary journey, remember that managing diverticulitis is an ongoing process. Staying informed, being mindful of dietary choices, and adapting as needed are key to maintaining health and comfort. This cookbook is a tool to help you on this path, providing guidance, inspiration, and practical solutions.

Managing diverticulitis through diet involves both understanding and adaptation. With thoughtful planning, informed choices, and a variety of delicious recipes, you can maintain a balanced and enjoyable diet that supports digestive health and overall well-being.

Embrace the journey with optimism and curiosity, and let this cookbook be a helpful companion in achieving a balanced and symptom-free lifestyle.

THANK YOU